Theosophy and Yoga

Also in this series:

Theosophy and the Search for Happiness
Texts by Moon Laramie and Annie Besant

Art and Theosophy
Texts by Martin Firrell and A.L. Pogosky

Theosophy and Esoteric Christianity
*Texts by Isis Resende, R. Heber Newton
& Franz Hartmann*

Forthcoming:

Theosophy and Social Justice
*Texts by Dr. Barbara B. Hebert, William Quan Judge
& Annie Besant*

Theosophy and Clairvoyance
Texts by Kurt Leland and C.W. Leadbeater

The Purpose of Theosophy
Texts by Petra Meyer and Patience Sinnett

Theosophy & Yoga

Texts by
Jenny Baker
& Annie Besant

martin firrell company
MODERN THEOSOPHY

First published in 2019 by Martin Firrell Company Ltd.
10 Queen Street Place, London EC4R 1AG, United Kingdom.

ISBN 978-1-912622-15-3

Design © Copyright Martin Firrell Company 2019.
Introduction © Copyright Moon Laramie 2019.
Essay © Copyright Jenny Baker 2019.

All rights reserved. No part of this publication may be reproduced, stored in or introduced into a retrieval system, or transmitted, in any form, or by any means (electronic, mechanical, photocopying, recording or otherwise) without the prior written consent of the publisher.

This book is sold subject to the condition that it shall not, by way of trade or otherwise, be lent, re-sold, hired out, or otherwise circulated without the publisher's prior consent in any form of binding or cover other than that in which it is published and without a similar condition including this condition being imposed on the subsequent purchaser.

Text is set in Baskerville, 12pt on 18pt.

Baskerville is a serif typeface designed in 1754 by John Baskerville (1706–1775) in Birmingham, England. Compared to earlier typeface designs, Baskerville increased the contrast between thick and thin strokes. Serifs were made sharper and more tapered, and the axis of rounded letters was placed in a more vertical position. The curved strokes were made more circular in shape, and the characters became more regular.

Baskerville is categorised as a transitional typeface between classical typefaces and high contrast modern faces. Of his own typeface, John Baskerville wrote,'Having been an early admirer of the beauty of letters, I became insensibly desirous of contributing to the perfection of them. I formed to myself ideas of greater accuracy than had yet appeared, and had endeavoured to produce a set of types according to what I conceived to be their true proportion.'

Introduction
by Moon Laramie

In April 1891, the theosophist Robert Bowen interviewed H.P. Blavatsky on the best approach to the study of theosophy. Her comments were published as a pamphlet in 1932 by Bowen's son, P. G. B. Bowen, under the title *Madame Blavatsky on How to Study Theosophy*. In it Blavatsky states, 'The True Student of The Secret Doctrine is a Jnana Yogi, and this Path of Yoga is the True Path for the Western student. It is to provide him with sign posts on that Path that The Secret Doctrine has been written.'

In this volume of the *Modern Theosophy* series, Jenny Baker, President of the Theosophical Society in England and Annie Besant, former International President of the Theosophical Society, each consider the connections between yoga and the theosophical tradition.

Jenny Baker explores how theosophy and yoga can guide the student on the path to self-realisation. She examines the way in which the two traditions are based on an understanding of the essential oneness of all life. It is through this understanding that greater self-realisation can be attained: 'The writers of the Upanishads used meditation as the chief means of obtaining transcendental knowledge. They used the name Brahman to describe the Absolute, and man's innermost identical self as Atman. Therefore the true meaning of yoga (union) is the realisation that Atman and Brahman are one.'

As Jenny Baker observes, the individual's search for meaning is a search for the true self, the inner being, the divine nature. It is through inner peace and stillness that this supreme self is revealed. In *An Introduction to Yoga*, Annie Besant writes that 'the Self in you is the same as the Self Universal… If you realise the unity of the Self amid the diversities of the Not-Self, then Yoga will not seem an impossible thing to you.' She suggests that far from retreating from the world, one should see it as an aid to self-realisation: 'The world is meant for the unfolding of the Self: why should you then seek to run away from it?' This is underlined by the theosophical concept that spiritual evolution is a learning process involving repeated earthly incarnations.

In his *Occult Glossary*, Gottfried de Purucker defines yoga as 'the attaining of union or at-oneness with the divine spiritual-essence within a man'. It is this divine spiritual-essence that Jenny Baker suggests 'lies unchanged behind the movements of the mind and is the constant light of our awareness'. Yoga, Annie Besant argues, is 'an applied science' which enables the individual to attain union with divine spiritual-essence through the 'unfolding of the whole consciousness of man on every plane, in every world'.

The Hindu sage Patanjali pointed out how 'one may, by individual, unaided, positive effort, lift the mind from its debased servitude to the emotions and the senses'.[1] This is an essential aspect of theosophy and yoga. Both traditions explore the importance of distinguishing between what is 'real' and what is 'unreal' - what should be the true focus of the mind and what is mere distraction. As Annie Besant explains, the world is full of 'forms that are illusory' and daily events are simply 'a dance of shadows'. This is echoed in Jenny Baker's observation that 'all that is impermanent is unreal.'

In his pamphlet *True and False Yoga*, Arthur Wells suggests that true yoga 'aims at providing a perfect body for the perfect Soul - the *mens sana in corpore sano* in the highest sense of the words'. Perhaps this dual aim of both yoga and theosophy is best summed up in Katherine Tingley's book *Theosophy: the Path of the Mystic*, cited by Jenny Baker. According to Tingley, 'Man must discover his own inner nature, his Real Self by his own efforts. To listen to his higher Self which is ever ready to help, there must be harmony of mind, soul and body.' Through dedicated practice, theosophy and yoga make such harmony an attainable outcome for us all.

1. *An Introduction to the Study of Yoga Aphorisms of Patanjali*
   G.C. Williams, Theosophical Publishing House 1933, first published in *The New California* theosophical magazine.

Jenny Baker

Jenny Baker is the President of the Theosophical Society in England (TSE). She has been a yoga teacher for more than 35 years and runs classes for people with multiple sclerosis and ME.

She joined the Theosophical Society in 1981 after attending a yoga weekend at Tekels Park, Camberley where she was initially introduced to theosophy and its concepts. She was particularly struck by the first object of the Theosophical Society - to form a nucleus of the Universal Brotherhood of Humanity without distinction of race, creed, sex, caste or colour. She was interested in the similarities between theosophy and yoga and decided to join the society immediately.

In 2005, she became a director of the annual English theosophical summer school. She was elected President of the TSE in 2015. During her time as president, the TSE hosted an International Conference on Annie Besant in 2017.

Jenny Baker has lectured on a range of topics including *The True Meaning of Brotherhood* and *Achieving Equilibrium Through Yoga*. She has led workshops on Yoga Nidra Relaxation. She cites H.P. Blavatsky's *The Voice of the Silence* as one of her major influences due to its relationship with the sacred texts of the Upanishads and the Bhagavad Gita. In a recent interview she said that she found a home in theosophy because 'its objects are very like my own philosophy of life'. Jenny Baker lives in south London, England.

Self-realisation through
Yoga and Theosophy
by Jenny Baker (2019)

'Self-realisation', 'yoga' and 'theosophy' are three very powerful words. There are many books written about all of these subjects so putting them together in one short text could be considered to be somewhat ambitious! The aim of this essay is to provide a flavour of all three and this may be an incentive for you to study them in greater detail. We'll begin with a brief introduction to each of them.

Our first word is 'self-realisation'. What exactly do we mean by 'self-realisation'? To answer this we need to understand what we mean by 'self' and why we need to realise this self. Many people through the centuries have wondered and asked themselves such questions as: 'Who am I?' The temple of Apollo at Delphi stated, 'Man know thyself.' We need to be able to distinguish between what is real and what is unreal. Until we have done that we will never be able to realise our true selves.

The second word is 'yoga'. What exactly do we mean by 'yoga'? There are many forms of yoga and how can we find the right one, which will lead us to the knowledge of our true selves? We will be looking at several different forms of yoga in this text.

Our final word is 'theosophy' which is often called divine wisdom. Like yoga it is a huge subject that requires a good deal of study. What we need to understand is how theosophy can guide us towards self-realisation.

Both yoga and theosophy are ancient traditions and in many ways they are comparable and compatible. I like to think of yoga as a form of theosophy and of theosophy as a part of the yoga tradition. They both have the oneness of life as their basis.

Part One: What Do We Mean by Self-realisation?

First, let's consider self-realisation. In the introduction to his autobiography, Gandhi says, 'What I want to achieve; what I have been striving and pining to achieve these thirty years is self-realisation; to see God face-to-face; to attain moksha[1]. I live and move and have my being in pursuit of this goal. All that I do in the way of speaking and writing, and all my ventures in the political field are directed to this same end.' Gandhi identifies self-realisation with spiritual salvation, which in Sanskrit is called moksha. This was his supreme goal in life; the goal that transcends both life and death. This is the goal revealed in the ancient scriptures of the East, the Upanishads and the Bhagavad Gita, to name just two of them.

Eastern philosophy states that the presence of our supreme self is revealed in a well-established state of inner peace and stillness which is made possible by minimising our desires for the things of the world.

The path to truth is man's greatest challenge. Gandhi confesses, 'I worship God as Truth only. I have not yet found Him, but I am seeking after Him and I am prepared to sacrifice the things dearest to me in pursuit of this quest. Even if the sacrifice demanded be my very life, I hope I may be prepared to give it.'

It is not only Gandhi's example that we could follow. Over the ages there have been many saints, sages, mystics and gurus from all religions and philosophies who have shown the way to a realisation of the God within.

There are also different names for self-realisation. Some call it enlightenment. Hindus refer to it as samadhi and Buddhists as nirvana. Yet others think of it as liberation or transcendence or Christ-consciousness or even the Kingdom of Heaven. But whatever name we give to our goal, what we seek is beyond, and greater than, our normal everyday existence.

When mankind starts to understand that there is more to life than material possessions, he starts to ponder on the meaning of life. Perhaps even asking questions such as: 'Why am I here?' 'What am I doing with my life?' 'Why am I still not satisfied with my life even though I have all my creature comforts and should be happy?'

Man realises that there is something missing from his life but often cannot put a name to it. He starts a search for that missing part of his life through religion, New Age cults, yoga and even theosophy. The search is for the true self, the inner being, the divine nature, that which never dies but is eternal; call it God, Christ, the Absolute, Krishna or innermost consciousness.

St Augustine wrote, 'Our hearts are ever restless until they find their rest in Thee.' Spiritual traditions all over the world recognise this restlessness. The Buddha also spoke of our restless hearts in his Four Noble Truths.

In the first truth, the experience of restlessness is described as sorrow, grief or frustration. In the second truth, the Buddha identifies the cause of that experience as the craving for what we do not have or are not. In the third, he says that the rest we seek is called nirvana, and in the fourth he affirms the existence of a path to that rest.

All spiritual traditions offer sets of guidelines; a route map to help us follow our chosen path to our destination. In the New Testament of the Bible, the Sermon on the Mount is just such a set of guidelines.

In the Hindu tradition there are the texts of the Upanishads and the Bhagavad Gita, which set us on the right path. Other traditions give us *The Dhammapada*,[2] *The Tao Te Ching*[3] and theosophy offers us three books, *At the Feet of the Master*, *Light on the Path* and *The Voice of the Silence*.

P. G. Bowen, in his booklet *The True Occult Path*, says there are two paths; an outer path and an inner one but it is only the inner path that leads to the truth, the Divine Wisdom.

In one of the Degrees of Freemasonry, the candidate is told that he must 'plunge in all humility into the mysteries and glorious depths of his own inmost being if he would win the Light he seeks, for each must find that hidden glory for himself, as all the Children of the Light have found it'.

Aldous Huxley, in *The Perennial Philosophy*, talks of 'a divine Reality, substantial to the world of things and lives and minds; the psychology that finds in the Soul something similar to or even identical with divine reality; the ethic that places man's final end in the knowledge of the immanent and transcendental Ground of all being.'

Rudiments of the perennial philosophy may be found among the traditional lore of primitive peoples in every religion of the world. In its fully developed form, the perennial philosophy has a place in each of the higher religions.

So far we have seen that there are many paths towards the goal of realising one's true self. But how would a yogi or a yogini start on his or her path to the truth?

Part Two: The Search for Self-realisation through the Practices and Philosophies of Yoga.

We know that yoga is very old, dating possibly to the period of the Rig Veda, about 3000BC or even earlier. The hymns contained in the Vedas were written by the sages or seers (also called Rishis or forest dwellers). They saw the truth behind manifest existence and revealed to ordinary men the luminous reality beyond all spiritual darkness. These Vedic seers won their sacred visions by their own hard work, their austerities and their deep impulse towards spiritual enlightenment.

The last section of the Vedas is called the Upanishads. These sacred books are ours to study and Madame Blavatsky says in her *Collected Writings*, 'that the Upanishads destroy ignorance and lead those who study them to spiritual liberation.' The writers of the Upanishads used meditation as the chief means of obtaining transcendental knowledge. They used the name Brahman to describe the Absolute, and man's innermost identical self as Atman. Therefore the true meaning of yoga (union) is the realisation that Atman and

Brahman are one. The Mundaka Upanishad says, 'the Atman is not reached by the weak, or the careless, or those who practise wrong austerity; but the wise who strive in the right way and lead their soul into the dwelling of Brahman. Having reached that place supreme, the seers find joy in wisdom, their souls have fulfilment, their passions have gone and they have peace. Filled with devotion, they have found the Spirit of All and gone into the All.'

Studying the Bhagavad Gita is another way for the aspirant to start on his path to self-realisation. The Lord's Song dates from between the 5th and 4th Centuries BC and forms an integral part of the great epic poem, well loved by Hindus, the Mahabharata.

The Bhagavad Gita is divided into 18 chapters and describes three different forms of yoga. These are Karma Yoga, Bhakti Yoga and Jnana Yoga; different paths to the same goal. Let us look at these in more detail.

Karma Yoga is the yoga of disinterested action. Bhakti Yoga is the yoga of love and devotion. Jnana Yoga is the yoga of knowledge. Then lastly there is Raja Yoga, to some the only relevant yoga.

It is the path of meditation which requires self-control, poise and tranquillity. All other yogas lead to Raja Yoga, as can be realised from studying the Bhagavad Gita where there are numerous mentions of meditation.

For instance, in chapter 17, verse 16 we read: 'Quietness of mind, silence, self-harmony, loving kindness and a pure heart; this is the harmony of the mind.'

In Chapter 18, verse 35 we read the following: 'When in the yoga of holy contemplation, the movements of the mind and of the breath of life are in a harmony of peace, there is a steadiness, and that steadiness is pure.'

The classical yoga of Patanjali is also known as Raja Yoga. Patanjali codified the yoga practices of his time. This yoga represents the climax of a long development of yogic techniques. Scholars think that Patanjali lived in the 2nd Century AD but nothing else is known about him. It is reasonable to assume that he was a great yoga authority, possibly the head of a school in which study was regarded as an important aspect of spiritual practice. In composing his sutras, he availed himself of existing works. He appears to have been a compiler rather than an originator.

He divides his yoga into eight parts known as limbs. These are:

(1)   *Yama*- self-restraint
(2)   *Niyama*- self-discipline
(3)   *Asana*- posture
(4)   *Pranayama*- breath control
(5)   *Pratyhara*- control of the senses
(6)   *Dharana*- concentration
(7)   *Dhyana*- meditation
(8)   *Samadhi*- contemplation.

The first two are moral codes and the next three are physical disciplines. These five can be practised together and naturally lead to the last three which are mental disciplines. For anyone striving for self-realisation the first two, Yama and Niyama, are particularly important because these provide moral guidelines without which self-realisation is not possible.

Yama is translated as meaning self-restraint. There are five yamas which deal with how we connect with other people and our responsibilities towards them. There are also five Niyamas, which means self-discipline, and they deal with our conduct towards ourselves.

The first Yama is Ahimsa, translated as non-violence. It means not doing any harm to others in thought, word or deed. We achieve this by adopting an attitude of kindness and helpfulness towards others and by having no desire to cause pain in any way and by asking at the end of the day, 'have I done anything to hurt anyone or been unkind today?'

This is the rule by which Mahatma Gandhi lived. Ahimsa is not easy to achieve. One has to be forever watchful over thoughts. Following a single unkind thought can easily be translated into a more damaging word and an even more harmful action. Be therefore ever watchful and aware of what you are thinking, speaking and doing every waking moment of the day and you will obtain Ahimsa.

The next Yama is Satya which translates as non-falsehood in the negative sense and truthfulness in the positive sense. This means not saying what we know to be untrue. The yogi should start by being true to himself and to his highest principles. A yogi should never justify a falsehood but be true in thought, word and deed.

Then comes Asteya which means non-stealing or to put it positively, honesty and uprightness. As well as not stealing other people's property, it also means not coveting what others have because coveting leads to dissatisfaction and envy. It is also possible to steal others words and ideas and pass them off as your own. A yogi should try to live an honest and upright life, desire-less of material possessions which do not give contentment.

The fourth Yama is Brahmacharya meaning non-sensuality. It can also be thought to mean self-restraint especially in sexual matters. The literal translation of Brahmacharya is: 'A life of holiness or religious study.' Ernest Wood[4] translates it as 'simple conduct'. It is probably best to think of it as temperance and self-control in all things such as eating, relationships, movement, emotional expression and in thought. The key words here are temperance, moderation and gentleness.

The last Yama is Aparigraha meaning non-acquisitiveness. It means not to be greedy or avaricious and not to hoard or collect. It could also be thought of as not accepting things one has not worked for or not accepting favours. By following Aparigraha, life becomes simple and discontent disappears. The important thing to consider is not how much one has but to use what one has to the best for oneself and others. It is well worth studying and even meditating on these five Yamas for they are closely linked. Achieving perfection in one will naturally lead to all the others.

Together these Yamas constitute the Great Vow that must be practised irrespective of place, time, circumstance or personal status. These moral attitudes are meant to bring our instinctual life under control. Moral integrity is an indispensable prerequisite of successful yoga practice.

We move onto the five Niyamas or self-restraints also known as observances.

The first one is Saucha meaning cleanliness or purity. It can be thought of in two ways: outer cleanliness or purity and inner cleanliness or purity. Outer cleanliness is keeping the physical body bathed, eating a good diet and breathing fresh air. Inner purity is achieved by concentration and meditation and by having a mind free from thoughts that corrupt or debase. Ultimately the personality in its highest aspect must be so pure that it mirrors the light of the transcendental self without distortion.

The second one is Santosha or contentment. This is a virtue that is diametrically opposed to our modern consumer mentality which is driven by the need to acquire ever more to fill the vacuum within. Contentment is an expression of renunciation, the voluntary sacrifice of what is destined to be taken from us at death. Santosha also means being able to experience success or failure, pleasure or sorrow with unshakeable equanimity and serenity.

The third Niyama is Tapas, meaning austerity. It is a self-discipline that gives the ability to withstand such things as hunger, thirst, prolonged periods of immobility, fasting, extreme heat or cold. It does not mean self-torture as practised by some fakirs or yogis in India. Practice of willpower develops strength of character, moral courage, a well-disciplined body and a balanced mind.

Number four is Swadhyaya. This is self-study and involves delving into the hidden meaning of the sacred texts. The purpose of Swadhyaya is not intellectual learning but absorption of the ancient wisdom. It is the meditative pondering of truths of the sages and seers who have traversed those remote regions where the mind cannot follow and only the heart receives and is changed. It also means studying oneself and one's progress towards spirituality.

The last Niyama is Ishwara-pranidhana. Translated as devotion to the Lord (Ishwara), it means opening one's heart to the transcendental being, the true self within. It is surrender to one's highest self. Practically, we can think of it as accepting the hand of God or a supreme director in every aspect of life. It is an acceptance of all experience without resentment. It means seeing the good in all things and is a dedication of all actions to the divinity within.

If we follow these ten moral codes to the best of our ability, we will surely be on the path to self-realisation, for they lead us directly to the last three limbs of Patanjali's Classical Yoga which are concentration, meditation and eventually Samadhi. Before we move on, I ought to mention

Mantra Yoga. This is the repetition of mantras or sacred sounds, either out loud or mentally. The repetition of various mantras can bring about a change of consciousness. Mantra Yoga uses vibration as a vehicle of transcendence and is one of the oldest forms of yoga coming from the time of the Vedas (3000BC). The best known mantra is OM.

Mantras can be used as magical tools but are also employed in spiritual contexts as instruments of empowerment. Mantras aid the aspirant's search for identification with the transcendental reality.

Part Three: Theosophy as a Pathway to Self-realisation

Like yoga, theosophy is ancient and derives from the ancient Stanzas of Dzyan which are of unknown origin. *The Key to Theosophy*, written by Madame Blavatsky, has this to say about reality: 'Remember the practically universal teaching of the two kinds of conscious existence: the terrestrial and the spiritual. The latter must be considered real from the very fact that it is inhabited by the eternal, changeless and immortal Monad.' Later she tells the enquirer, 'Your spiritual 'I' is immortal.'

Blavatsky also says, 'We assert that the Divine Spark in man, being one and identical in its essence with the Universal Spirit, our Spiritual Self, is practically omniscient, but that it cannot manifest its knowledge owing to the impediments of matter... Now the more these impediments are removed, the more fully can the inner Self manifest on this plane.'

In *The Key to Theosophy*, Madame Blavatsky quotes from *The Theosophist*. 'Let everyman be a revelation unto himself. Let once man's immortal spirit take possession of the temple of his body, drive out the money-changers and every unclean thing, and his own divine humanity will redeem him, for when he is thus at one with himself he will know the builder of the temple.'

The motto of the Theosophical Society is: 'There is no religion higher than truth.' Some think it should say: 'There is no Dharma higher than truth.' What is meant by 'truth'? It is that the spirit of man, our true self, is perfect and is not different from the supreme spiritual force that underlies the universe. 'Myself is the self of all,' is the realisation of one who knows the ultimate truth. Our true nature is not our personality, the face we offer to the world, but the divine wealth of peace, bliss and knowledge that resides deep within us.

We seem to be creatures of opposites for we are controlled by time yet our roots are in eternity. We seem to be limited in body and mind yet our spirit is infinite. We seem to be individuals whose personalities are known to ourselves and others yet within us all there is a divine centre that is one, universal, pure consciousness and absolute.

So how can we distinguish between what is real and what is unreal? All that is impermanent is unreal. This means everything that is subject to change, from the largest mountain to the smallest grain of sand, cannot be considered real. What is real is that which never changes, our divine consciousness, and this is what we seek to realise. The true self lies unchanged behind the movements of the mind and is the constant light of our awareness.

I mentioned the three books that offer guidance on the path. They are *At the Feet of the Master*, *Light on the Path* and *The Voice of the Silence*.

These three guide books address different aspects of our journey. They are inevitably similar because they are concerned with the same experience. *At the Feet of the Master* is preparatory, dealing with what comes first. It answers the question: 'How do I prepare to walk the path?'

Light on the Path is progressive, being concerned with what the path itself is like. It answers the question: 'What will I find as I walk the path?'

The Voice of the Silence is cumulative, leading up to what comes at the end of the path. It answers the question: 'Where does the path lead?' *At the Feet of the Master* was written by Jiddu Krishnamurti[5] as a child while under nightly instruction by the Mahatmas. At the end of each nightly session, the teacher summarised the basic points of the instruction in a few sentences. Each morning, when the boy awoke, he would write down what he remembered of the previous night's teaching. The writings were gathered together and published in 1910 as *At the Feet of the Master* under the pen name 'Alcyone'.

The four parts of the book set out in modern language the four ancient qualifications for entering the path. They are 1: Discrimination or right choosing. 2: Desirelessness or right viewing. 3: Good conduct or right action. 4: Love or right response.

Light on the Path was first published in 1885. It was written down by Mabel Collins, a prolific author of the 19th Century. The book has three levels of material. At its core are 30 short aphoristic and often enigmatic 'rules', each of which is an instruction or order to do something. The second level of the book consists of amplifications of the 30 rules and the third level is a series of more prosaic notes or commentaries.

The Voice of the Silence was published by Madame Blavatsky in 1889, four years after *Light on the Path*. It consists of 316 verses ranging in length from several words to a few sentences. The verses are in three fragments which Blavatsky says are extracts from a longer work called, *The Book of the Golden Precepts*, another spiritual guidebook.

All three fragments are about the journey a pilgrim makes on the path of spiritual development and are focused on what lies at the end of the path.

Another book worth studying is *The Technique of the Spiritual Life* by Clara Codd[6] who was imprisoned as a suffragette. Codd was librarian and General Secretary at the London Theosophical Society. The book was first published in 1958.

There is another useful book, *Theosophy: the Path of the Mystic* written by Katherine Tingley[7] and published in 1922. Tingley was born in Massachusetts in 1847 and was introduced to theosophy by William Quan Judge. When he died in 1896, she took over as head of the Theosophical Society in America. She lectured in the United States and around the world. To her, theosophy was never 'a system of sterile thought' but remained always 'a light, a teacher, a companion ever calling to compassionate action, ever urging to higher things'.

The following are some helpful quotes from her book:

'Man cannot find his true place in the great scheme of human life until he has ennobled his nature with the consciousness of his divinity. That is the message of theosophy.'

'The aim of theosophy is that each may come to know himself better; that there may be spiritual rounding out of the character and the life. To rise in the strength of his divine heritage there comes a clearing of the mind, a lifting of the veil that hides the truth.'

'Human nature is dual, a battle between higher and lower self, angel and demon. When the higher immortal part dominates there is knowledge and peace. When the lower rules all the dark despairing elements of human life rush in upon the unguarded soul.'

'Man must discover his own inner nature, his Real Self by his own efforts. To listen to his higher Self which is ever ready to help, there must be harmony of mind, soul and body.'

So how does man discover his higher self? Tingley suggests keeping positive, having a steady joy in one's heart and by having right feeling and thought. She also says it is by meditation, by dwelling in brotherhood and by having compassion for all. She says we must be warriors and not be discouraged.

We must have faith and free ourselves from pre-conceived ideas. We should harmonise thought and action and have pure motives for those actions. We should surrender our lower nature, our selfish, lustful nature to the God within us. Wisdom, she suggests, comes from the performance of duty.

There are three key ways, Tingley says, by which we can reach an understanding of our self. These are self-study, self-analysis and self-control. The inner nature seeks perfection which is the truth.

Calling forth this inner divine self illuminates the mind and brings us to the highest spiritual discernment, to knowledge of the higher self.

Madame Blavatsky offers the following advice on this subject: 'Success does not come without effort. Progress is made step by step and each step gained by heroic effort. Be hopeful then, not despairing. With each morning's awakening, try to live through the day in harmony with the Higher Self. Try, is the battle-cry taught by the Teachers to each pupil. Naught else is expected of you. One who does his best does all that can be asked.'[8]

In *The Song Celestial*, Edward Arnold writes, 'Never the spirit was born; the spirit shall cease to be never. Never was time it was not: End and beginning are dreams. Birthless and deathless and changeless remaineth the spirit. Death hath not touched it at all.'

In verse 19 of *The Voice of the Silence*, Madame Blavatsky writes, 'Saith the Great Law: In order to become the KNOWER OF ALL-SELF, thou hast first of Self to be the knower. To reach the knowledge of that Self, thou hast to give up self to non-self, being to non-being, and then thou canst repose between the wings of the Great Bird. Aye, sweet is the rest between the wings of that which is not born, nor dies, but is the AUM[9] throughout eternal ages.'

Self-realisation can be achieved by any of several forms of yoga. The one to choose will be the one that best suits your temperament and personality. So if you like doing things then Karma Yoga will be best for you. If you are a devotional type of person then Bhakti Yoga is the one for you. If you like using your intellect then Gnana is what you should study. If you like chanting then Mantra Yoga will be your path to self-realisation. Raja Yoga is for those keen on meditation as a way to enlightenment.

Theosophy uses some parts of all the above mentioned forms of yoga as it encourages us to be compassionate, to work for others, to be loving and humble. Theosophy tells us to discriminate between that which is real and that which is unreal and between what is right and what is wrong. It shows us how to use the inner path and to learn to listen to our inner voice. Ultimately, both yoga and theosophy teach the oneness of all life.

1. Moksha, also called vimoksha, vimukti and mukti, is a term in Hinduism, Buddhism, Jainism and Sikhism which refers to various forms of emancipation, enlightenment, liberation and release.

2. The Dhammapada is a collection of sayings of the Buddha in verse form.

3. The Tao Te Ching, also known as Lao Tzu or Laozi, is a Chinese text from the 6th Century BC, traditionally credited to

the sage Laozi. It is a fundamental text for both philosophical and religious Taoism.

4. Ernest Egerton Wood (18 August 1883 - 17 September 1965) was a noted English yogi, theosophist, Sanskrit scholar and author.

5. Jiddu Krishnamurti (12 May 1895 - 17 February 1986) was an Indian philosopher, speaker and writer. His writings explored the nature of the mind, meditation, human relationships and the potential for radical change in society.

6. Clara Margaret Codd (10 October 1876 - 3 April 1971) was a British writer, suffragette and theosophist. In 1908, she was arrested for her suffragette activities outside the House of Commons and sentenced to a month in prison. Her later work as a theosophist included two years service at the Theosophical Society's headquarters in Adyar, India. Codd continued to lecture around the world, on behalf of the society, for the rest of her life.

7. Katherine Tingley (6 July 1847 - 11 July 1929) was a social worker and prominent theosophist. She became the leader of the American Section of the Theosophical Society, succeeding William Quan Judge in 1896.

8. From *Stars and Stones on the Path A Practical Manual for Aspirants to Theosophy*, compiled and edited by Dr C.A. Bartzokas.

9. The syllable 'om' is composed of the three sounds a-u-m (the vowels 'a' and 'u' create the compound sound 'o' in Sanskrit) mystically symbolising the essence of the entire universe.

Annie Besant

Annie Besant was born in London on 1 October 1847. She was a women's rights activist, supporter of Irish independence, socialist, author and was president of the Theosophical Society from 1907 until her death in 1933. In 1867, she married Frank Besant, a clergyman, and they had two children. However, her criticism of his political and religious views led to their legal separation in 1873. She then became an active member of the National Secular Society (NSS). In 1877, she helped publish a book, *Fruits of Philosophy* by Charles Knowlton, the American birth control campaigner. The ensuing scandal put her in the public spotlight. Besant was a prolific writer and initially wrote a weekly column in *The National Reformer*. In her articles she argued for Irish home rule and a secular state in Britain. Later Besant became involved with social justice campaigns, including the London match girls strike of 1888. She was a prominent speaker for the Fabian Society and the Marxist Social Democratic Federation. In 1889, she was asked to write a review for *The Pall Mall Gazette* on *The Secret Doctrine*, the seminal work by Helena Petrovna Blavatsky. She sought an interview with its author and met

Blavatsky in Paris. Blavatsky was one of the founder members of the theosophical movement along with Henry Steel Olcott and William Quan Judge. The society was set up to promote the comparative study of philosophy, religion and science. The society described itself as 'an unsectarian body of seekers after Truth, who endeavour to promote Brotherhood and strive to serve humanity'.

Besant joined the Theosophical Society and soon became a leading lecturer and author on theosophical subjects. She published a number of books including *Thought Forms* (with C.W. Leadbeater) in 1901 and *Esoteric Christianity* in 1905. While president of the Theosophical Society, Besant was based at its headquarters in Adyar, India. She became involved in the struggle for Indian self-determination and helped launch the Home Rule League in 1914. In the late 1920s, Besant travelled to the United States with her protégé Jiddu Krishnamurti, who she hailed as the new World Teacher and incarnation of Buddha. Although Krishnamurti distanced himself from theosophy in 1929, Besant remained loyal to him. After her death, Krishnamurti, Aldous Huxley, Guido

Ferrando, and Rosalind Rajagopal built the Besant Hill School of Happy Valley in her honour. Besant's many pamphlets include *The Gospel of Christianity and the Gospel of Freethought* (1883), *Life, Death, and Immortality* (1886), *Why I Do Not Believe in God* (1887), and *Theosophy and the Search for Happiness* (1918).

The Nature of Yoga
by Annie Besant (1907)
*One of four lectures given at the 32nd anniversary
of the Theosophical Society, Benares, India*

Foreword

These lectures are intended to give an outline of Yoga, in order to prepare the student to take up, for practical purposes, the *Sutras of Patanjali*, the chief treatise on Yoga. I have on hand, with my friend Bhagavan Das as collaborator, a translation of these Sutras, with Vyasa's commentary, and a further commentary and elucidation written in the light of Theosophy. To prepare the student for the mastering of that more difficult task, these lectures were designed; hence the many references to Patanjali. They may, however, also serve to give to the ordinary lay reader some idea of the Science of sciences, and perhaps to allure a few towards its study.

The Nature of Yoga

In this first discourse we shall concern ourselves with the gaining of a general idea of the subject of Yoga, seeking its place in nature, its own character, its object in human evolution.

The Meaning of the Universe

Let us, first of all, ask ourselves, looking at the world around us, what it is that the history of the world signifies. When we read history, what does the history tell us? It seems to be a moving panorama of people and events, but it is really only a dance of shadows; the people are shadows, not realities, the kings and statesmen, the ministers and armies; and the events - the battles and revolutions, the rises and falls of States - are the most shadow-like dance of all. Even if the historian tries to go deeper, if he deals with economic conditions, with social organisations, with the study of the tendencies of the currents of thought, even then he is in the midst of shadows, the illusory shadows cast by unseen realities. This world is full of forms that are illusory, and the values are all wrong, the proportions are out of focus. The things which a man of the world thinks valuable, a spiritual man must cast aside as worthless. The diamonds of the world, with their glare and glitter in the rays of the outside sun, are mere fragments of broken glass to the man of knowledge. The crown of the King, the sceptre of the Emperor, the triumph of earthly power, are less than nothing to the man who has had one glimpse of the majesty of the Self. What is, then, real? What is truly valuable? Our answer will be very different from the answer given by the man of the world.

'The universe exists for the sake of the Self.' Not for what the outer world can give, not for control over the objects of desires, not for the sake even of beauty or pleasure, does the Great Architect plan and build His worlds. He has filled them with objects, beautiful and pleasure-giving. The great arch of the sky above, the mountains with snow-clad peaks, the valleys soft with verdure and fragrant with blossoms, the oceans with their vast depths, their surface now calm as a lake, now tossing in fury, they all exist, not for the objects themselves, but for their value to the Self. Not for themselves, because they are anything in themselves, but that the purpose of the Self may be served, and his manifestations made possible.

The world, with all its beauty, its happiness and suffering, its joys and pains, is planned with the utmost ingenuity, in order that the powers of the Self may be shown forth in manifestation. From the fire-mist to the Logos, all exist for the sake of the Self. The lowest grain of dust, the mightiest Deva in his heavenly regions, the plant that grows out of sight in the nook of a mountain, the star that shines aloft over us - all these exist in order that the fragments of the one Self, embodied in countless forms, may realise their own identity, and manifest the powers of the Self through the matter that envelops them.

There is but one Self in the lowliest dust and the loftiest Deva. 'Mamamsaha, My portion, a portion of My Self,' says Sri Krishna, are all these Jivatmas,[1] all these living spirits. For them the universe exists; for them the sun shines, and the waves roll, and the winds blow, and the rain falls, that the Self may know himself as manifested in matter, as embodied in the universe.

The Unfolding of Consciousness

One of those pregnant and significant ideas which Theosophy scatters so lavishly around is this - that the same scale is repeated over and over again, the same succession of events in larger or smaller cycles. If you understand one cycle, you understand the whole. The same laws by which a solar system is built go to the building up of the system of man. The laws by which the Self unfolds his powers in the universe, from the fire-mist up to the Logos, are the same laws of consciousness which repeat themselves in the universe of man. If you understand them in the one, you can equally understand them in the other. Grasp them in the small, and the large is revealed to you. Grasp them in the large, and the small becomes intelligible to you.

The great unfolding from the stone to the God goes on through millions of years, through aeons of time. But the long unfolding that takes place in the universe, takes place in a shorter time-cycle within the limit of humanity, and this in a cycle so brief that it seems as nothing beside the longer one. Within a still briefer cycle a similar unfolding takes place in the individual - rapidly, swiftly, with all the force of its past behind it. These forces that manifest and unveil themselves in evolution are cumulative in their power. Embodied in the stone, in the mineral world, they grow and put out a little more of strength, and in the mineral world accomplish their unfolding. Then they become too strong for the mineral, and press on into the vegetable world. There they unfold more and more of their divinity, until they become too mighty for the vegetable, and become animal.

Expanding within and gaining experiences from the animal, they again overflow the limits of the animal, and appear as the human. In the human being they still grow and accumulate with ever-increasing force, and exert greater pressure against the barrier; and then out of the human, they press into the super-human. This last process of evolution is called 'Yoga'.

Coming to the individual. The man of our own globe has behind him his long evolution in other chains than ours - this same evolution through mineral to vegetable, through vegetable to animal, through animal to man, and then from our last dwelling-place in the lunar orb on to this terrene globe that we call the earth. Our evolution here has all the force of the last evolution in it, and hence, when we come to this shortest cycle of evolution which is called Yoga, the man has behind him the whole of the forces accumulated in his human evolution, and it is the accumulation of these forces which enables him to make the passage so rapidly. We must connect our Yoga with the evolution of consciousness everywhere, else we shall not understand it at all; for the laws of evolution of consciousness in a universe are exactly the same as the laws of Yoga, and the principles whereby consciousness unfolds itself in the great evolution of humanity are the same principles that we take in Yoga and deliberately apply to the more rapid unfolding of our own consciousness. So that Yoga, when it is definitely begun, is not a new thing, as some people imagine.

The whole evolution is one in its essence. The succession is the same, the sequences identical. Whether you are thinking of the unfolding of consciousness in the universe, or in the human race, or in the individual, you can study the laws of the whole, and in Yoga you learn to apply those same laws to your own consciousness rationally and definitely. All the laws are one, however different in their stages of manifestation.

If you look at Yoga in this light, then this Yoga, which seemed so alien and so far off will begin to wear a familiar face, and come to you in a garb not wholly strange.

As you study the unfolding of consciousness, and the corresponding evolution of form, it will not seem so strange that from man you should pass on to superman, transcending the barrier of humanity, and finding yourself in the region where divinity becomes more manifest.

The Oneness of the Self

The Self in you is the same as the Self Universal. Whatever powers are manifested throughout the world, those powers exist in germ, in latency, in you. He, the Supreme, does not evolve. In Him there are no additions or subtractions. His portions, the Jivatmas, are as Himself, and they only unfold their powers in matter as conditions around them draw those powers forth. If you realise the unity of the Self amid the diversities of the Not-Self, then Yoga will not seem an impossible thing to you.

The Quickening of the Process of Self-unfoldment

Educated and thoughtful men and women you already are; already you have climbed up that long ladder which separates the present outer form of the Deity in you from His form in the dust. The manifested Deity sleeps in the mineral and the stone. He becomes more and more unfolded in vegetables and animals, and lastly in man He has reached what appears as His culmination to ordinary men. Having done so much, shall you not do more? With the consciousness so far unfolded, does it seem impossible that it should unfold in the future into the divine? As you realise that the laws of the evolution of form and of the unfolding of consciousness in the universe and man are the same, and that it is through these law's that the Yogi brings out his hidden powers, then you will understand also that it is not necessary to go into the mountain or into the desert, to hide yourself in a cave or a forest, in order that the union with the Self may be obtained - He who is within you and without you. Sometimes for a special purpose seclusion may be useful. It may be well at times to retire temporarily from the busy haunts of men. But in the universe planned by Isvara,[2] in order that the powers of the Self may be brought out - there is your best field for Yoga, planned with Divine wisdom and sagacity. The world is meant for the unfolding of the Self: why should you then seek to run away from it? Look at Shri Krishna Himself in that great Upanishad of Yoga, the Bhagavad-Gita. He spoke it out on a battlefield, and not on a mountain peak. He spoke it to a Kshattriya ready to fight, and not to a Brahmana quietly retired from the world. The Kurukshetra of the world is the field of Yoga. They who cannot face the world have not the strength to face the difficulties of Yoga practice. If the outer world out-wearies your powers, how do you expect to conquer the difficulties of the inner life? If you cannot climb over the little troubles of the world, how can you hope to climb over the difficulties that a Yogi has to scale? Those men blunder, who think that running away from the world is the road to victory, and that peace can be found only in certain localities. As a matter of fact, you have practised Yoga unconsciously in the past, even before your Self-consciousness had separated itself, was aware of itself, and knew itself to be different, in temporary matters at least, from all the others that surround it. And that is the first idea that you should take up and hold firmly: Yoga is only a quickened process of the ordinary unfolding of consciousness. Yoga may then be defined as the 'rational application of the laws of the unfolding of consciousness in an individual case.' That is what is meant by the methods of Yoga. You study the laws of the unfolding of consciousness in the universe, you then apply them to a special case - and that case is your own. You cannot apply them to another. They must be self-applied. That is the definite principle to grasp. So we must add one more word to our definition: 'Yoga is the rational application of the laws of the unfolding of consciousness, self-applied in an individual case.'

Yoga is a Science

Next: Yoga is a science. That is the second thing to grasp. Yoga is a science, and not a vague, dreamy drifting or imagining. It is an applied science, a systematised collection of laws applied to bring about a definite end. It takes up the laws of psychology, applicable to the unfolding of the whole consciousness of man on every plane, in every world, and applies those rationally in a particular case. This rational application of the laws of unfolding consciousness acts exactly on the same principles that you see applied around you every day in other departments of science.

You know, by looking at the world around you, how enormously the intelligence of man, cooperating with nature, may quicken 'natural' processes, and the working of intelligence is as 'natural' as anything else. We make this distinction, and practically it is a real one, between 'rational' and 'natural' growth, because human intelligence can guide the working of natural laws; and when we come to deal with Yoga, we are in the same department of applied science as, let us say, is the scientific farmer or gardener, when he applies the natural laws of selection to breeding. The farmer or gardener cannot transcend the laws of nature, nor can he work against them. He has no other laws of nature to work with save the universal laws by which nature is evolving forms around us, and yet he does in a few years what nature takes, perhaps, hundreds of thousands of years to do. And how? By applying human intelligence to choose the laws that serve him, and to neutralise the laws that hinder. He brings the divine intelligence in man to utilise the divine powers in nature, that are working for general rather than for particular ends.

Take the breeder of pigeons. Out of the blue rock pigeon he develops the pouter, or the fantail; he chooses out, generation after generation, the forms that show most strongly the peculiarity that he wishes to develop. He mates such birds together, takes every favouring circumstance into consideration, and selects again and again, and so on and on, till the peculiarity that he wants to establish has become a well-marked feature. Remove his controlling intelligence, leave the birds to themselves, and they revert to the ancestral type.

Or take the case of the gardener. Out of the wild rose of the hedge has been evolved every rose of the garden. Many-petalled roses are but the result of the scientific culture of the five-petalled rose of the hedge-row, the wild product of nature. A gardener who chooses the pollen from one plant and places it on the carpels of another is simply doing deliberately what is done every day by the bee and the fly. But he chooses his plants, and he chooses those that have the qualities he wants intensified, and from those again he chooses those that show the desired qualities still more clearly, until he has produced a flower so different from the original stock that only by tracing it back can you tell the stock whence it sprang.

So is it in the application of the laws of psychology that we call Yoga. Systematised knowledge of the unfolding of consciousness applied to the individualised self, that is Yoga. As I have just said, it is by the world that consciousness has been unfolded, and the world is admirably planned by the Logos for this unfolding of consciousness; hence the would-be Yogi, choosing out his objects and applying his laws, finds in the world exactly the things he wants to make his practice of Yoga a real, a vital thing, a quickening process for the knowledge of the Self. There are many laws. You can choose those which you require, you can evade those you do not require, you can utilise those you need, and thus you can bring about the result that nature, without that application of human intelligence, cannot so swiftly effect.

Take it, then, that Yoga is within your reach, within your powers, and that even some of the lower practices of Yoga, some of the simpler applications of the laws of the unfolding of consciousness to yourself, will benefit you in this world as well as in all others. For you are really merely quickening your growth, your unfolding, taking advantage of the powers nature puts within your hands, and deliberately eliminating the conditions which would not help you in your work, but rather hinder your march forward. If you see it in that light, it seems to me that Yoga will be to you a far more real, practical thing, than it is when you merely read some fragments about it taken from Sanskrit books, and often mistranslated into English, and you will begin to feel that to be a Yogi is not necessarily a thing for a life far off, an incarnation far removed from the present one.

Man a Duality

Some of the terms used in Yoga are necessarily to be known. For Yoga takes man for a special purpose and studies him for a special end, and, therefore, only troubles itself about two great facts regarding man, mind and body. First, he is a unit, a unit of consciousness. That is a point to be definitely grasped. There is only one of him in each set of envelopes, and sometimes the theosophist has to revise his ideas about man when he begins this practical line. Theosophy, quite usefully and rightly, for the understanding of the human constitution, divides man into many parts and pieces. We talk of physical, astral, mental, etc. Or we talk about Sthula-sarira, Sukshama-sarira, Karana-sarira, and so on. Sometimes we divide man into Anna-maya-kosa, Prana-maya-kosa, Mano-maya-kosa, etc. We divide man into so many pieces, in order to study him thoroughly, that we can hardly find the man because of the pieces. This is, so to say, for the study of human anatomy and physiology.

But Yoga is practical and psychological. I am not complaining of the various subdivisions of other systems. They are necessary for the purpose of those systems. But Yoga, for its practical purposes, considers man simply as a duality, a mind and body, a unit of consciousness in a set of envelopes. This is not the duality of the Self and the Not-Self. For in Yoga, 'Self' includes consciousness plus such matter as it cannot distinguish from itself, and Not- Self is only the matter it can put aside.

Man is not pure Self, pure consciousness, Samvid. That is an abstraction. In the concrete universe there are always the Self and his sheaths, however tenuous the latter may be, so that a unit of consciousness is inseparable from matter, and a Jivatmi, or Monad, is invariably consciousness plus matter.

In order that this may come out clearly, two terms are used in Yoga as constituting man - Prana and Pradhana, life-breath and matter. Prana is not only the life-breath of the body, but the totality of the life-forces of the universe, or, in other words, the life-side of the universe.

'I am Prana,' says Indra.[3] Prana here means the totality of the life-forces. They are taken as consciousness, mind. Pradhana is the term used for matter. Body, or the opposite of mind, means for the

Yogi in practice so much of the appropriated matter of the outer world as he is able to put away from himself, to distinguish from his own consciousness.

This division is very significant and useful, if you can catch clearly hold of the root idea. Of course, looking at the thing from beginning to end, you will see Prana, the great Life, the great Self, always present in all, and you will see the envelopes, the bodies, the sheaths, present at the different stages, taking different forms; but from the standpoint of yogic practice, that is called Prana, or Self, with which the man identifies himself for the time, including every sheath of matter from which the man is unable to separate himself in consciousness. That unit, to the yogi, is the Self, so that it is a changing quantity. As he drops off one sheath after another and says: 'That is not myself,' he is coming nearer and nearer to his highest point, to consciousness in a single film, in a single atom of matter, a Monad. For all practical purposes of Yoga, the man, the working, conscious man, is so much of him as he cannot separate from the matter enclosing him, or with which he is connected. Only that is body which the man is able to put aside and say:

'This is not I, but mine.' We find we have a whole series of terms in Yoga which may be repeated over and over again. All the states of mind exist on every plane, says Vyasa,[4] and this way of dealing with man enables the same significant words, as we shall see in a moment, to be used over and over again, with an ever-subtler connotation; they all become relative, and are equally true at each stage of evolution.

Now it is quite clear that, so far as many of us are concerned, the physical body is the only thing of which we can say: 'It is not myself'; so that, in the practice of Yoga at first, for you, all the words that would be used in it to describe the states of consciousness, the states of mind, would deal with the waking consciousness in the body as the lowest state, and, rising up from that, all the words would be relative terms, implying a distinct and recognisable state of the mind in relation to that which is the lowest. In order to know how you shall begin to apply to yourselves the various terms used to describe the states of mind, you must carefully analyse your own consciousness, and find out how much of it is really consciousness, and how much is matter so closely appropriated that you cannot separate it from yourself.

States of Mind

Let us take it in detail. Four states of consciousness are spoken of amongst us. Waking, or Jagrat; the 'dream' consciousness or Svapna; the 'deep sleep' consciousness, or Sushupti; and the state beyond that, called Turiya. How are those related to the body?

Jagrat is the ordinary waking consciousness, that you and I are using at the present time. If our consciousness works in the subtle, or astral, body and is able to impress its experiences upon the brain, it is called Svapna, or in English, dream consciousness; it is more vivid and real than the Jagrat state. When working in the subtler form, the mental body, it is not able to impress its experiences on the brain, it is called Sushupti, or deep sleep consciousness; then the mind is working on its own contents, not on outer objects. But if it has so far separated itself from connection with the brain, that it cannot be readily recalled by outer means, then it is called Turiya, a lofty state of trance. These four states, when correlated to the four planes, represent a much unfolded consciousness. Jagrat is related to the physical; Svapna to the astral; Sushupti to the mental; and Turiya to the buddhic. When passing from one world to another, we should use these words to designate the consciousness working under the conditions of each world. But the same words are repeated in the books of Yoga with a different context. There the difficulty occurs, if we have not learned their relative nature. Svapna is not the same for all, nor is sushupti the same for everyone.

Above all the word Samadhi, to be explained in a moment, is used in different ways and different senses. How then are we to find our way in this apparent tangle? By knowing the state which is the starting-point, and then the sequence will always be the same. All of you are familiar with the waking consciousness in the physical body. You can find four states even in that, if you analyse it, and a similar sequence of the states of the mind is found on every plane.

How to distinguish them, then? Let us take the waking consciousness, and try to see the four states in that. Suppose I take up a book and read it. I read the words; my eyes are related to the outer physical consciousness. That is the Jagrat state, I go behind the words to the meaning of the words. I have passed from the waking state of the physical plane into the Svapna state of waking consciousness, that sees through the outer form, seeking the inner life. I pass from this to the mind of the writer; here the mind touches the mind; it is the waking consciousness in its Sushupti state. If I pass from this contact and enter the very mind of the writer, and live in that man's mind, then I have reached the Turiya state of the waking consciousness.

Take another illustration. I look at my watch; I am in Jagrat. I close my eyes and make an image of the watch; I am in Svapna. I call together many ideas of many watches, and reach the ideal watch; I am in Sushupti. I pass to the idea of time in the abstract; I am in Turiya. But all these are stages in the physical plane consciousness; I have not left the body.

In this way, you can make states of mind intelligible and real, instead of mere words.

Samadhi

Some other important words which recur from time to time in the Yoga Sutras, need to be understood, though there are no exact English equivalents. As they must be used to avoid clumsy circumlocutions, it is necessary to explain them. It is said: 'Yoga is Samadhi.' Samadhi is a state in which the consciousness is so dissociated from the body that the latter remains insensible. It is a state of trance, in which the mind is fully self-conscious, though the body is insensitive, and from which the mind returns to the body with the experiences it has had in the super-physical state, remembering them when again immersed in the physical brain. Samadhi for any one person is relative to his waking consciousness, but implies insensitiveness of the body. If an ordinary person throws himself into trance and is active on the astral plane, his Samadhi is on the astral. If his consciousness is functioning in the mental plane, his Samadhi is there. The man who can so withdraw from the body as to leave it insensitive, while his mind is fully self-conscious, can practise Samadhi. The phrase 'Yoga is Samadhi' covers facts of the highest significance and greatest instruction. Suppose you are only able to reach the astral world when you are asleep, your consciousness there is, as we have seen, in the svapna state. But as you slowly unfold your powers, the astral forms begin to intrude upon your waking physical consciousness, until they appear as distinctly as do physical forms, and thus become objects of your waking consciousness. The astral world then, for you, no longer belongs to the svapna consciousness, but to the jagrat; you have taken two worlds within the scope of your jagrat consciousness - the physical and the astral worlds - and the mental world is in your svapna consciousness. Your 'body' is then the physical and the astral bodies taken together. As you go on, the mental plane begins to similarly intrude itself, and the physical, astral and mental all come within your waking consciousness; all these are, then, your jagrat world. These three worlds form but one world to you; their three corresponding bodies but one body, that perceives and acts. The three bodies of the ordinary man have become one body for the Yogi. If under these conditions you want to see only one world at a time, you must fix your attention on it, and thus focus it. You can, in that state of enlarged waking, concentrate your attention on the physical and see it; then the astral and mental will appear hazy. So you can focus your attention on the astral and see it; then the physical and the mental, being out of focus, will appear dim. You will easily understand this, if you remember that, in this hall, I may focus my sight in the middle of the hall, when the pillars on both sides will appear indistinctly. Or I may concentrate my attention on a pillar and see it distinctly, but I then see you only vaguely at the same time. It is a change of focus, not a change of body. Remember that all which you can put aside as not yourself is the body of the Yogi, and hence, as you go higher, the lower bodies form but a single body, and the consciousness in that sheath of matter which it still cannot throw away, that becomes the man.

'Yoga is Samadhi.' It is the power to withdraw from all that you know as body, and to concentrate yourself within. That is Samadhi. No ordinary means will then call you back to the world that you have left. This will also explain to you the phrase in *The Secret Doctrine* that the Adept 'begins his Samadhi on the atmic plane. 'When an Indian Yogi in Samadhi, discovered in a forest by some ignorant and brutal Englishmen, was so violently ill-used that he returned to his tortured body, only to leave it again at once by death. When a Jivanmukta[5] enters into Samadhi, he begins it on the atmic plane. All planes below the atmic are one plane for him. He begins his Samadhi on a plane to which the mere man cannot rise. He begins it on the atmic plane, and thence rises stage by stage to the higher cosmic planes. The same word, Samadhi, is used to describe the states of the consciousness, whether it rises above the physical into the astral, as in the self-induced trance of an ordinary man, or, as in the case of a Jivanmukta, when, the consciousness being already centred in the fifth, or atmic, plane, it rises to the higher planes of a larger world.

The Literature of Yoga

Unfortunately for non-Sanskrit-knowing people, the literature of Yoga is not largely available in English. The general teachings of Yoga are to be found in the Upanishads and the Bhagavad Gita, those, in many translations, are within your reach but they are general, not special; they give you the main principles but do not tell you about the methods in any detailed way. Even in the Bhagavad Gita, while you are told to make sacrifices, to become indifferent, and so on, it is all of the nature of moral precept, absolutely necessary indeed, but still not telling you how to reach the conditions put before you. The special literature of Yoga is, first of all, many of the minor Upanishads, 'the hundred-and-eight' as they are called. Then comes the enormous mass of literature called the Tantras. These books have an evil significance in the ordinary English ear, but not quite rightly. The Tantras are very useful books, very valuable and instructive; all occult science is to be found in them. But they are divisible into three classes; those that deal with white magic, those that deal with black magic, and those that deal with what we may call grey magic, a mixture of the two. Now 'magic' is the word which covers the methods of deliberately bringing about super-normal physical states by the action of the will.

A high tension of the nerves, brought on by anxiety or disease, leads to ordinary hysteria, emotional and foolish. A similarly high tension, brought about by the will, renders a man sensitive to super-physical vibrations. Going to sleep has no significance, but going into Samadhi is a priceless power. The process is largely the same, but one is due to ordinary conditions, the other to the action of the trained will.

The Yogi is the man who has learned the power of the will, and knows how to use it to bring about foreseen and foredetermined results. This knowledge has ever been called magic; it is the name of the 'Great Science' of the past, the one Great Science, to which only the word 'great' was given in the past. The Tantras contain the whole of that; the occult side of man and nature, the means whereby discoveries may be made, the principles whereby the man may recreate himself, all these are in the Tantras. The difficulty is that without a teacher they are very dangerous, and again and again a man trying to practise the tantric methods without a teacher makes himself very ill. So the Tantras have got a bad name both in the West and here in India.

A good many of the American 'occult' books now sold are scraps of the Tantras which have been translated. One difficulty is that these tantric works often use the name of a bodily organ to represent an astral or mental centre. There is some reason in that, because all the centres are connected with each other from body to body; but no reliable teacher would set his pupil to work on the bodily organs, until he had some control over the higher centres, and had carefully purified the physical body. Knowing the one helps you to know the other, and the teacher who has been through it all can place his pupil on the right path; but if you take up these words, which are all physical, and do not know to what the physical word is applied, then you will only become very confused, and may injure yourselves. For instance, in one of the sutras it says that if you meditate on a certain part of the tongue you will obtain astral sight. That means that if you meditate on the pituitary body, just over this part of the tongue, astral sight will be opened. The particular word used to refer to a centre has a correspondence in the physical body, and the word is often applied to the physical organs when the other is meant. This is what is called a 'blind' and it is intended to keep the people away from dangerous practices in the books that are published; people may meditate on that part of their tongues all their lives without anything coming of it; but if they think upon the corresponding centre in the body, a good deal - much harm - may come of it. 'Meditate on the navel' it is also said. This means the solar plexus, for there is a close connection between the two. But to meditate on that is to incur the danger of a serious nervous disorder, almost impossible to cure. All who know how many people in India suffer through these practices, ill understood, recognise that it is not wise to plunge into them without some one to tell you what they mean, and what may be safely practised and what not.

The other part of the Yoga literature is a small book called The Sutras of Patanjali. That is available, but I am afraid that few are able to make much of it by themselves. In the first place, to elucidate the sutras, which are simply headings, there is a great deal of commentary in Sanskrit, only partially translated. And even the commentaries have this peculiarity, that all the most difficult words are merely repeated, not explained, so that the student is not much enlightened.

Some Definitions

There are a few words, constantly recurring, which need brief definitions, in order to avoid confusion; they are: unfolding, evolution, spirituality, psychism, yoga, and mysticism.

'Unfolding' always refers to consciousness, 'evolution' to forms. Evolution, according to Herbert Spencer,[6] is the homogeneous becoming the heterogeneous, the simple becoming complex. But there is no growth and no perfectioning for Spirit, for consciousness; it is all there and always, and all that can happen to it is to turn itself outwards instead of remaining being turned inwards. The God in you cannot evolve, but He may show forth His powers through matter that He has appropriated for the purpose, and the matter evolves to serve Him. He Himself only manifests what He is. And on that, many a saying of the great mystics may come to your mind: 'Become,' says St. Ambrose,[7] 'what you are' - a paradoxical phrase, but one that sums up a great truth: become in outer manifestation that which you are in inner reality. That is the object of the whole process of Yoga.

'Spirituality' is the realisation of the One.

'Psychism' is the manifestation of intelligence through any material vehicle. 'Yoga' is the seeking of union by the intellect, a science; 'Mysticism' is the seeking of the same union by emotion.

See the mystic. He fixes his mind on the object of devotion; he loses self-consciousness, and passes into a rapture of love and adoration, leaving all external ideas, wrapped in the object of his love, and a great surge of emotion sweeps him up to God. He does not know how he has reached that lofty state. He is conscious only of God and his love for Him. Here is the rapture of the mystic, the triumph of the saint.

The Yogi does not work like that. Step after step, he realises what he is doing. He works by science and not by emotion, so that any who do not care for science, finding it dull and dry, are not at present unfolding that part of their nature which will find its best help in the practice of Yoga. The Yogi may use devotion as a means. This comes out very plainly in Patanjali. He has given many means whereby Yoga may be followed, and, curiously, 'devotion to Ishvara' is one of several means. There comes out the spirit of the scientific thinker.

Devotion to Ishvara is not for him an end in itself, but a means to an end - the concentration of the mind. You see there at once the difference of spirit. Devotion to Ishvara is the path of the mystic. He attains communion by that. Devotion to lshvara as a means of concentrating the mind is the scientific way in which the Yogi regards devotion. No number of words would have brought out the difference of spirit between Yoga and Mysticism as well as this. The one looks upon devotion to Ishvara as a way of reaching the Beloved; the other looks upon it as a means of reaching concentration. To the mystic, God, in Himself is the object of search, delight in Him is the reason for approaching Him, union with Him in consciousness is his goal; but to the Yogi, fixing the attention on God is merely an effective way of concentrating the mind. In the one, devotion is used to obtain an end; in the other, God is seen as the end, and is reached directly by rapture.

God without and God within

Now that leads us to the next point, the relation of God without to God within. To the Yogi, who is the very type of Hindu thought, there is no definite proof of God save the witness of the Self within to His existence, and his idea of finding the proof of God is that you should strip away from your consciousness all limitations, and thus reach the stage where you have pure consciousness - save a veil of the thin nirvanic matter. Then you know that God is. So you read in the Upanishad: 'Whose only proof is the witness of the Self.' This is very different from western methods of thought, which try to demonstrate God by a process of argument. The Hindu will tell you that you cannot demonstrate God by any argument or reasoning; He is above and beyond reasoning, and although the reason may guide you on the way, it will not prove to demonstration that God is. The only way you can know Him is by diving into yourself. There you will find Him, and know that He is without as well as within you; and Yoga is a system that enables you to get rid of everything from consciousness that is not God, save that one veil of the nirvanic atom, and so to know that God is, with an unshakeable certainty of conviction. To the Hindu that inner conviction is the only thing worthy to be called 'faith' and this gives you the reason why faith is said to be beyond reason, and so is often confused with credulity. Faith is beyond reason, because it is the testimony of the Self to himself, that conviction of existence as Self, of which reason is only one of the outer manifestations, and the only true faith is that inner conviction, which no argument can either strengthen or weaken, of the innermost Self of you, that of which alone you are entirely sure. It is the aim of Yoga to enable you to reach that Self constantly, not by a sudden glimpse of intuition, but steadily, unshakeably, and unchangeably, and when that Self is reached, then the question: 'Is there a God?' can never again come into the human mind.

Changes of Consciousness and Vibrations of Matter

Now it is necessary to understand something about that consciousness which is your Self, and about the matter which is the envelope of consciousness, but which the Self so often identifies with himself. The great characteristic of consciousness is change, with a foundation of certainty that it is. The consciousness of existence never changes, but beyond this all is change, and only by the changes does consciousness become Self-consciousness. Consciousness is an ever-changing thing circling round one idea that never changes - Self-existence. The consciousness itself is not changed by any change of position or place. It only changes its states within itself.

In matter, every change of state is brought about by change of place. A change of consciousness is a change of state; a change of matter is a change of place. Moreover, every change of state in consciousness is related to vibrations of matter in its vehicle. When matter is examined, we find three fundamental qualities - rhythm, mobility, stability - sattva, rajas, tamas. Sattva is rhythm, vibration. It is more than rajas, or mobility. It is a regulated movement, a swinging from one side to the other over a definite distance, a length of wave, a vibration.

The question is often put: 'How can things in such different categories as Matter and Spirit affect each other? Can we bridge that great gulf which Tyndall said can never be crossed?' Yes, the Indian has crossed it, or rather, has shown that there is no gulf. To the Indian, Matter and Spirit are not only the two phases of the One, but by a subtle analysis of the relation between consciousness and matter, he sees that in every universe the Logos imposes upon matter a certain definite relation of rhythms, every vibration of matter corresponding to a change in consciousness. There is no change in consciousness, however subtle, that has not appropriated to it a vibration in matter; there is no vibration in matter, however swift or delicate, which has not correlated to it a certain change in consciousness. That is the first great work of the Logos, which the Hindu scriptures trace out in the building of the atom, the Tanmatra, 'the measure of That', the measure of consciousness. He who is consciousness imposes on His material the answer to every change in consciousness, and that is an infinite number of vibrations. So that between the Self and its sheaths there is this invariable relation: the change in consciousness and the vibration of matter, and vice versa. That makes it possible for the Self to know the Not-self.

These correspondences are utilised in Raja Yoga and Hatha Yoga, the Kingly Yoga and the Yoga of Resolve. The Raja Yoga seeks to control the changes in consciousness, and by this control to rule the material vehicles. The Hatha Yoga seeks to control the vibrations of matter, and by this control to evoke the desired changes in consciousness. The weak point in Hatha Yoga is that action on this line cannot reach beyond the astral plane, and the great strain imposed on the comparatively intractable matter of the physical plane sometimes leads to atrophy of the very organs, the activity of which is necessary for effecting the changes in consciousness that would be useful. The Hatha Yogi gains control over the bodily organs with which the waking consciousness no longer concerns itself, having relinquished them to its lower part, the 'subconsciousness'. This is often useful as regards the prevention of disease, but serves no higher purpose. When he begins to work on the brain centres, connected with ordinary consciousness, and still more when he touches those connected with the super-consciousness, he enters a dangerous region, and is more likely to paralyse than to evolve.

That relation alone it is which makes matter cognisable; the change in the thinker is answered by a change outside, and his answer to it, and the change in it that he makes by his answer, rearrange again the matter of the body which is his envelope. Hence the rhythmic changes in matter are rightly called its cognisability. Matter may be known by consciousness, because of this unchanging relation between the two sides of the manifested Logos who is one, and the Self becomes aware of changes within Himself, and thus of those of the external world to which those changes are related.

Mind

What is mind? From the yogic standpoint it is simply the individualised consciousness, the whole of it, the whole of your consciousness including your activities - which the western psychologist puts outside mind. Only on the basis of eastern psychology is Yoga possible. How shall we describe this individualised consciousness? First, it is aware of things. Becoming aware of them, it desires them. Desiring them, it tries to attain them. So we have the three aspects of consciousness - intelligence, desire, activity. On the physical plane, activity predominates, although desire and thought are present. On the astral plane, desire predominates, and thought and activity are subject to desire. On the mental plane, intelligence is the dominant note, desire and activity are subject to it. Go to the buddhic plane, and cognition, as pure reason, predominates, and so on. Each quality is present all the time, but one predominates. So with the matter that belongs to them. In your combinations of matter you get rhythmic, active, or stable ones; and according to the combinations of matter in your bodies will be the conditions of the activity of the whole of these in consciousness. To practise Yoga you must build your bodies of the rhythmic combinations, with activity and inertia less apparent. The Yogi wants to make his body match his mind.

Stages of Mind

The mind has five stages, Patanjali tells us, and Vyasa comments that 'these stages of mind are on every plane.' The first stage is the stage in which the mind is flung about, the Kshipta stage: it is the butterfly mind, the early stage of humanity, or, in man, the mind of the child, darting constantly from one object to another. It corresponds to activity on the physical plane. The next is the confused stage, Mudha, equivalent to the stage of the youth, swayed by emotions, bewildered by them; he begins to feel he is ignorant - a state beyond the fickleness of the child - a characteristic state, corresponding to activity in the astral world. Then comes the state of preoccupation, or infatuation, Vikshipta, the state of the man possessed by an idea, love, ambition, or what not. He is no longer a confused youth, but a man with a clear aim, and an idea possesses him. It may be either the fixed idea of the madman, or the fixed idea which makes the hero or the saint; but in any case he is possessed by the idea. The quality of the idea, its truth or falsehood, makes the difference between the maniac and the martyr.

Maniac or martyr, he is under the spell of a fixed idea. No reasoning avails against it. If he has assured himself that he is made of glass, no amount of argument will convince him to the contrary. He will always regard himself as being as brittle as glass. That is a fixed idea which is false. But there is a fixed idea which makes the hero and the martyr. For some great truth dearer than life is everything thrown aside. He is possessed by it, dominated by it, and he goes to death gladly for it. That state is said to be approaching Yoga, for such a man is becoming concentrated, even if only possessed by one idea. This stage corresponds to activity on the lower mental plane. Where the man possesses the idea, instead of being possessed by it, that one-pointed state of the mind, called Ekagrata in Sanskrit, is the fourth stage. He is a mature man, ready for the true life. When the man has gone through life dominated by one idea, then he is approaching Yoga; he is getting rid of the grip of the world, and is beyond its allurements. But when he possesses that which before possessed him, then he has become fit for Yoga, and begins the training which makes his progress rapid. This stage corresponds to activity on the higher mental plane.

Out of this fourth stage, or Ekagrata, arises the fifth stage, Niruddha or Self-controlled. When the man not only possesses one idea, but, rising above all ideas, chooses as he wills, takes or does not take according to the illumined Will, then he is Self-controlled, and can effectively practise Yoga. This stage corresponds to activity on the buddhic plane.

In the third stage, Vikshipta, where he is

possessed by the idea, he is learning Viveka, or discrimination between the outer and the inner, the real and the unreal. When he has learned the lesson of Viveka, then he advances a stage forward; and in Ekagrata he chooses one idea, the inner life; and as he fixes his mind on that idea he learns Vairagya, or dispassion. He rises above the desire to possess objects of enjoyment, belonging either to this or any other world. Then he advances towards the fifth stage - Self-controlled. In order to reach that he practises the six endowments, the Shatsamapatti. These six endowments have to do with the Will-aspect of consciousness, as the other two, Viveka and Vairagya, have to do with the cognition and activity aspects of it.

By a study of your own mind, you can find out how far you are ready to begin the definite practice of Yoga. Examine your mind in order to recognise these stages in yourselves. If you are in either of the two early stages, you are not ready for Yoga. The child and the youth are not ready to become Yogis, nor is the preoccupied man. But if you find yourself possessed by a single thought, you are nearly ready for Yoga; it leads to the next stage of one-pointedness, where you can choose your idea, and cling to it of your own will. Short is the step from that to the complete control, which can inhibit all motions of the mind. Having reached that stage, it is comparatively easy to pass into Samadhi.

Inward and Outward Turned Consciousness

Samadhi is of two kinds: one turned outward, one turned inward. The outward-turned consciousness is always first. You are in the stage of Samadhi belonging to the outward-turned waking consciousness, when you can pass beyond the objects to the principles which those objects manifest, when through the form you catch a glimpse of the life. Darwin was in this stage when he glimpsed the truth of evolution. That is the outward-turned Samadhi of the physical body.

This is technically the Samprajnata Samadhi, the 'Samadhi with consciousness', but to be better regarded, I think, as with the consciousness outward-turned, i.e. conscious of objects. When the object disappears, that is when consciousness draws itself away from the sheath by which those objects are seen, then comes the Asamprajnata Samadhi called the 'Samadhi without consciousness'. I prefer to call it the inward-turned consciousness, as it is by turning away from the outer that this stage is reached.

These two stages of Samadhi follow each other on every plane; the intense concentration on objects in the first stage, and the piercing thereby through the outer form to the underlying principle, are followed by the turning away of the consciousness from the sheath which has served its purpose, and its withdrawal into itself, i.e., into a sheath not yet recognised as a sheath. It is then for a while conscious only of itself and not of the outer world. Then comes the 'cloud', the dawning sense again of an outer, a dim sensing of 'something' other than itself; that again is followed by the functioning of the higher sheath and the recognition of the objects of the next higher plane, corresponding to that sheath. Hence the complete cycle is: Samprajnata Samadhi, Asamprajnata Samadhi, Megha (cloud), and then the Samprajnata Samadhi of the next plane, and so on.

The Cloud.

This term - in full, Dharma-Megha, cloud of righteousness, or of religion - is one which is very scantily explained by the commentators. In fact, the only explanation they give is that all the man's past karma of good gathers over him, and pours down upon him a rain of blessing. Let us see if we cannot find something more than this meagre interpretation.

The term 'cloud' in very often used in the mystic literature of the West; the 'Cloud on the Mount', the 'Cloud on the Sanctuary', the 'Cloud on the Mercy-Seat', are expressions familiar to the student. And the experience which they indicate is familiar to all mystics in its lower phases, and to some in its fullness. In its lower phases, it is the experience just noted, where the withdrawal of the consciousness into a sheath not yet recognised as a sheath is followed by the beginning of the functioning of that sheath, the first indication of which is the dim sensing of an outer. You feel as though surrounded by a dense mist, conscious that you are not alone, but unable to see. Be still; be patient; wait. Let your consciousness be in the attitude of suspense. Presently the cloud will thin, and first in glimpses, then in its full beauty, the vision of a higher plane will dawn on your entranced sight. This entrance into a higher plane will repeat itself again and again, until, your consciousness centred on the buddhic plane, and its splendours having disappeared as your consciousness withdraws even from that exquisite sheath, you find yourself in the true cloud, the cloud on the sanctuary, the cloud that veils the Holiest, that hides the vision of the Self. Then comes what seems to be the draining away of the very life, the letting go of the last hold on the tangible, the hanging in a void, the horror of great darkness, loneliness unspeakable. Endure, endure. Everything must go. 'Nothing out of the Eternal can help you.' God only shines out in the stillness; as says the Hebrew: 'Be still, and know that I am God.' In that silence a Voice shall be heard, the voice of the Self. In that stillness a Life shall be felt, the life of the Self. In that void a Fullness shall be revealed, the fullness of the Self. In that darkness a Light shall be seen, the glory of the Self. The cloud shall vanish, and the shining of the Self shall be made manifest. That which was a glimpse of a far-off majesty shall become a perpetual realisation, and, knowing the Self and your unity with it, you shall enter into the Peace that belongs to the Self alone.

1. In Hinduism and Jainism, a Jivatma is an individual soul.

2. Ishvara is a concept in Hinduism, with a wide range of meanings that depend on the era and the school of Hinduism. In ancient texts of Indian philosophy, depending on the context, Ishvara can mean supreme soul, ruler, lord, king, queen or husband. In medieval era Hindu texts, depending on the school of Hinduism, Ishvara means God, supreme being, personal god, or special self. In Shaivism and for many Hindus, Ishvara is synonymous with 'Shiva', sometimes as Maheshvara or Parameshvara meaning the 'supreme lord', or as an Ishta-deva (personal god). Similarly for Vaishnavists and many Hindus, it is synonymous with Vishnu. In traditional Bhakti movements, Ishvara is one or more deities of an individual's preference from Hinduism's polytheistic canon of deities. In modern sectarian movements such as Arya Samaj and Brahmoism, Ishvara takes the form of a monotheistic God. In the Yoga school of Hinduism, it is any 'personal deity' or 'spiritual inspiration'. In the Advaita Vedanta school, Ishvara is a monistic universal absolute that connects and is the oneness in everyone and everything.

3. Indra is a Vedic deity in Hinduism, a guardian deity in Buddhism, and the king of the highest heaven called Saudharmakalpa in Jainism. His mythologies and powers are similar to other Indo-European deities such as Jupiter, Perun, Perkūnas, Taranis, Zeus, and Thor. In the Vedas, Indra is the king of Svarga (heaven) and the Devas. He is the god of the heavens, lightning, thunder, storms, rains, river flows, and war. Indra is the deity referred to most often in the Rigveda.

4. Vyasa is the legendary author of the Mahabharata, Vedas and Puranas, some of the most important works in the Hindu tradition. He is also called Veda Vyāsa ('the one who classified the Vedas') or Krishna Dvaipāyana (referring to his dark complexion and birthplace). Vyasa is also considered to be one of the seven Chiranjivins (long-lived, or immortals) who are still in existence, according to Hindu tradition.

5. A jivan mukta is someone who, in the Advaita Vedanta philosophy of Hinduism, has gained and assimilated infinite and divine knowledge and power, and gained complete self-knowledge and self-realisation, attaining kaivalya or moksha (enlightenment and liberation). The individual is liberated with an inner sense of freedom while still living. This state is the aim of moksha in Advaita Vedanta, Yoga and other schools of Hinduism, and is referred to as Jivanmukti (liberation or enlightenment).

6. Herbert Spencer (27 April 1820 - 8 December 1903) was an English philosopher, biologist, anthropologist, sociologist, and prominent liberal political theorist of the Victorian era.

7. Aurelius Ambrosius (c. 340 - 397), better known in English as Ambrose, was a bishop of Milan who became one of the most influential ecclesiastical figures of the 4th Century. He was the Roman governor of Liguria and Emilia, headquartered in Milan, before being made bishop of Milan by popular acclamation in 374. Ambrose was one of the four original Doctors of the Church, and is the patron saint of Milan.

www.ingramcontent.com/pod-product-compliance
Lightning Source LLC
Chambersburg PA
CBHW021127080526
44587CB00012B/1173